G-gasm Method: The Ultimate Guide to the G-spot Orgasm

How to Have a Woman Experience 10, 20 or Even 50 Big O's Per Night.

G-gasm Method: The Ultimate Guide to the G-spot Orgasm
How to Have a Woman Experience 10, 20 or Even 50 Big O's Per Night.

By: Jani - Published by Bonnie's Gang Publishing, New York

Although based on actual experience, some events in this book have been fictionalized to protect the privacy of certain individuals.

Please consult your Doctor if you are pregnant, have had a caesarean, surgery or infections before trying the G-gasm Method. As with anything, use common sense.

Copyright 2006 Bonnie's Gang

All rights reserved. No part of this book may be reproduced, stored in a retrieval system, transmitted in electronic form, or any other means reproduced without the prior permission of Bonnie's Gang.

Bonnie's Gang Publishing

Please visit us at:
G-gasm.com

ISBN # 0-9762090-4-7

For the

1,767,397,107*

ladies that have

never experienced an orgasm.

*My very rough estimate

Forward

Sex with your lover is the fuel that keeps love burning hot. Love is not necessary for sex, however, the stronger the emotional connection is, the better the sexual experience happens to be. My goal is to invigorate all marriages and long-term relationships.

I am one of the few fortunate men in the world, who after 20+ years of marriage, can still say:

*I am glad that I married.
*I love my wife.
*My wife is my best friend.
*We still have great sex.

How many of you guys can honestly say those four statements? I bet not many. Guys this book is all about her – and how to please her sexually. I don't give a rat's ass about how horny you are. Learn how to please your lady … and she will make you the happiest guy on Earth.

Please visit www.G-gasm.com to share your thoughts, experiences and to help spread the word about the G-gasm Method.

Table of Contents

Foreplay – What are G-spots and G-gasms - page 6

First Base - Learning the G-spot – Page 12

Second Base - The G-gasm Method – Page 25

Third Base - Variations of the Method – Page 53

Home Run – The Best Part – Page 72

Email … We get email – Page 78

Guys A Warning! – Page 93

Foreplay

> "Pulling my sweetheart close to me, her hips reacting to the gentle tug ... my hand reaches up towards her soft shoulders, her head tilts ... my moist lips caress the skin under her ear ... she nudges me on ... I softly bite the area that joins her neck and shoulder, she places her hands around my shoulders ... our lips meet ..."

Before my current long-term relationship, of 20+ years, I was working the dating scene. I was in my mid 20's and during this period, all I was looking for in relationships were FB's – fuck buddies. I had no interest in any kind of long-term relationship – I just wanted to have some fun.

During this time, I met a FB named Gloria. Gloria was in her early 30's and horny as a Las Vegas slut. Neither one of us was looking for commitment. We could be open and honest, and often discussed our sexual play. Her clit was like a detonator; I would flick that little red marble with my tongue, until she exploded.

Gloria had been away, and I had been missing her while she was on her trip, and was eager to let her know how glad I was to have her back.

I invited Gloria to come over to my place for a visit. Everything was ready. I lit the candles, had a bottle of white wine on ice, some John Coltrane playing; the mood was set for some loving. Body oil, lube and a couple of vibrators crammed the bedside table drawer.

Before Gloria had left on her trip, her and I had talked about G-spots, and while she was away, I had read about and learned the secrets of mastering the G-spot. I had an idea – The G-gasm Method – and I wanted to share it with her.

Gloria was hot. She was not beautiful or anything, but she was sexy. When she walked down the street, heads tuned so fast I swear some of those guys got whiplash. But it was men and women both who turned to see her long brown hair and nice round ass. Her high heels made her even sexier. OK, maybe I have a little bit of a foot fetish, but the shoes she wore made her smoking hot.

Gloria arrived at my place around seven o'clock. I gently kissed her warm perfumed skin and thought of how beautiful she looked when I opened the door to greet her. Her black shirt stretched across her chest, contrasting sharply with her smooth soft milky white skin.

My arms encircled her as I leaned towards her; she raised her head to meet my willing lips. She parted her lips for my tongue; I explored her mouth insistently, yet gently. My hands slowly slid down her back until they rested on Gloria's wonderful ass. She raised her head and smiled at me, and I knew then that she wanted me as much as I wanted her.

As I poured her a glass of wine, Gloria stepped up from behind, and wrapped her arms around my waist; her hands trailed down past my belt buckle and teasingly clutched at my rising cock.

I set down my beer, and guided her to my bedroom, we sat down and I pulled her into my lap. We kissed deeply, while I ran my hands up and down her legs and body. Her light green eyes looked deeply into mine, and her face spread into a wicked, naughty grin. Without breaking eye contact, I pushed her legs apart, ran my hand up the inside of Gloria's thigh and squeezed her pussy firmly. Gloria gasped and trembled a bit as her breath grew shorter. Gloria bucked hard against my hand, but I teasingly withdrew it and continued to stroke the inside of her thighs. Every now and then, my finger would rub up against her clit and she would let out a soft moan.

She unbuttoned my shirt, and ran her long fingers over my chest; her red polished nails playfully flicked my nipples. Gloria gave me a seductive glance, slid off my lap and got on her knees between my legs. She knelt there for a minute, running her hands up and down my thighs, gazing at the outline of my bulging cock. She smiled and pressed me back to a reclining position. Her hands trailed down my chest across my waist as she unbuckled my belt and opened my pants. She unzipped me as I raised my hips and pushed my pants to the floor.

Gloria leaned in close, and ran her fingers along my engorged shaft. She playfully stroked and kissed the base of my cock, then worked her soft lips and tongue slowly and teasingly up my shaft. She took the head of my cock between her lips, and gently rolled her tongue around the rim. On every downward stroke, very slowly, she took more and more of me into her tender mouth. Gloria often sucked me until I squirted her in the mouth and was eager to take it all, but when she took her lips off me for a second to catch her breath, I lifted her to her feet and spun her on the bed next to me. Tonight, I had different plans.

I raised Gloria's blouse over her head, undid her bra and slipped it off exposing her breasts. Her nipples were pink and as hard as little pebbles. I unzipped her jeans, slipped them down over her ass and threw them to the floor.

I was tweaking and teasing her nipples, as I nibbled at them tenderly. Meanwhile, my other hand was massaging her crotch through her moist panties; she was getting extremely aroused.

We continued kissing, caressing and licking each other's bodies. We had already played with spanking; I tied Gloria's arms and hands to the bedposts. She was now face down and spread-eagled across the bed. Gloria thought I was going to smack her on the ass and the thought made her dripping wet with excitement.

I could not help smiling when Gloria thought she was about to get some spanking action. I have yet to find a woman who did not enjoy - that did not get off on a nice loving whack on the ass. Now, I am not talking about inflicting pain or anything – that is a completely different topic. What I am talking about is the act of lovingly spanking a beautiful bottom, which is not physical abuse.

I think it works both ways too. I have had a couple of ladies decide that a stiff slap to my bottom was what I needed to crank things up a notch or two or three. However, this is something we will explore at another time.

"You haven't spanked me for a long time...," Gloria whispered as she wiggled her butt up in the air.

It was very cute and cuddly. I have a theory, the butt, both nipples and the vagina are all somehow wired together. Touching, squeezing, pinching or kissing any one part causes a reaction in the other two. Something primordial about a spanking – big tough guy male whacking his woman to show her that he is the boss somehow gets the nipples erect and the pussy wet.

I gave Gloria a couple good hard smacks just to get her all warmed up and dribbling wet. We had been experimenting with a foam backed ping-pong paddle. Gloria was loud – I mean LOUD. She would produce, not just moaning, but actual screaming.

I yanked her panties aside and rubbed my stiff cock up and down and across her pussy, just barely grazing the lips with the head of my cock. She tried to shove her ass back toward me, in a vain effort to get my cock in her hot little hole.

"Oh does poor little Gloria want to be fucked? Do you?" I teased.

I put my knee up between Gloria's legs and buried it in her crotch, rotating and massaging her there. I felt her warm moisture leak out and run over my skin. I put my hand on her hot pussy and dipped a finger inside ... she was very, very wet..."Oh! Baby!" I smiled naughtily, reacting to her extreme readiness.

"Please fuck me … stick your cock in me," Gloria whispered.

"Don't worry, you're going to get fucked," I said with a cruel grin, "But I have other plans first."

She nodded meekly as I continued to play and toy with her pussy lips, spreading them apart and fingering her.

First Base

A guy goes to a supermarket and notices a beautiful blonde who waves at him and then says hello.

He is rather taken back, because he cannot place where he knows her from, so he says, "Do you know me?"

To which she replies, "I think you're the father of one of my kids."

Now he thinks back to the only time he has ever been unfaithful to his wife and says, "My God, are you the stripper from my bachelor party that I fucked on the pool table with all my buddies watching, while your partner whipped my ass with wet celery and then stuck a carrot up my ass?"

She said, "NOOOOO..., I'm your son's Math Teacher."

Guys and gals, you are about to learn a life changing sex Method. Sex will never be as it once was. Men, once you master this, she will be your sex slave forever.

This Method is so easy; anyone can master it and perform like a porn star. Once you, and the lucky woman you are trying the G-gasm Method on, find the right spot, she will be so happy she will be telling all her girlfriends. Then what are you going to do? You will have girls lining up at your bedroom door.

The G-gasm Method will make you a confident lover. You will make any woman multi orgasmic. You will learn the skills to please any and every woman. It doesn't matter who you are or what kind of person you are, when you try this Method, you will succeed and she will thank you for it. OK, 'thank you' is a very mild way of saying, "THAT WAS FAN-FUCKING-TASTIC!" You are about to learn how to give your lady the ultimate pleasure and satisfaction.

I am not a celebrity or a sex therapist. I am not a doctor so this book will not provide you with any form of medical jargon. You will not find a flow chart of the vagina or any type of medical advice that you could logically expect to find when you are speaking to a doctor. If you are looking for that kind of information, I am sorry, Yahoo "woman's vagina" – you will get all the info you need. There is not a doctor in the world that will teach you, what you are about to learn here.

I have never really kept track, but I have made love to (done, fucked, screwed ... whatever) over 50 women. I have no medical training but I can teach you plenty of things about a woman's body, her G-spot and the right way to stimulate it to create orgasm after mind blowing orgasm. The G-gasm Method is not hard to do once you know exactly where to find the G-spot, and how to fire it up correctly.

Attitude

Ok guys pay attention. I could write a whole book on this topic, there are extremely too many guys walking around with the wrong attitude. You are a man, so act like a man – be a man – don't be a girly-man.

Guys, you do not have to be debonair and sophisticated, you do not need any "moves," all you need is attitude - the right attitude, not the wrong attitude. There are ladies for all **men**, notice I emphasize men. Girls like: strong, weak, thin, husky – not fat, tall, short – well not too short, rugged, scrawny, young, old, you don't need perfect hair, perfect teeth, perfect skin, or a perfect body. In other words, unless you are a big fat disgusting slob with wind chimes dangling in your mouth disguised as teeth, there are girls out there for you.

Too many guys are walking around looking like they slept in a pile of dirty laundry. Groom yourself every day – shower, shave, trim your nose hairs and eyebrows, squeeze out those blackheads from your face, clip your nails and keep your hair clean and neat. When you are in a position to meet ladies – which is just about always – dress nice, and smell nice. Yeah, that's right, smell nice, put on some cologne – the ladies love that.

You need the right attitude. By attitude I mean your overall outlook and the manner in which you conduct yourself. Your feelings, your thoughts, the way you behave, your opinion of right and wrong and your way of thinking are all part of having the right attitude. Some attributes of the "right attitude," in no particular order of importance.

Smile a lot

Don't talk too much

Be a good listener

Be loyal to those that deserve your loyalty

Be clean and neat

Follow **your** traditions and values

Realize that getting there is 90% of the fun

Whatever you do – do it at 100%

It's **not** all about you

Be honest

Respect people that deserve respect

Try to help – especially when no one is looking

Be persistent

Dream – then plan

Are you going to do everything above all the time? No, but do get in the habit of having the right attitude, woman look for that in a man.

I am not a particularly good-looking guy, I'm about six feet tall and weigh 195 pounds. I have long light brown hair that is always clean and tied back in a ponytail. I have an acne-scarred face, that resembles the lunar surface, and when God was handing out noses, I thought he said roses – "I'll take the big red one in the corner," I said. My usual attire is jeans, boots and some kind of a black tee shirt. I try to follow my own advice above, and have the right attitude. I've never had a shortage of women, there were many times that I would be juggling 2 or 3 FB's at a time. Guys, you know how that works - while you are banging one girl, you tell her that the other one is a pig. When you are banging the "pig," you tell her the other one is a slut.

The average man believes a woman's body is like a whodunit mystery. When I started dating women, I was a dense dimwit. I thought the only thing I had to do was stick my dick in her pussy, jackhammer away as fast and hard as I could and we both would be happy. First one smoking a cigarette wins. Guess what? It does not work that way, not even close. I have learned a great deal about the female anatomy. I have figured out what makes them explode with orgasmic pleasure. Most men have no clue how to master satisfying a woman. But you my friend, are about to learn the secrets of the G-gasm Method.

Reading this, means you are curious about becoming a sexual superman. It is hard to believe that any man, even some kind of a Don Juan, could give a woman 50 G-gasms in one night! You can make it happen; this method works. I am offering you the guidance and knowledge needed to perform this Method. In time, your wife/girlfriend/lover/FB will believe you are a super stud in the bedroom.

What is a G-gasm?

Let us first define orgasm.

The meaning of life.

A discharge of neuromuscular tensions at the apex of sexual stimulation that is accompanied by the ejaculation of semen in men and by vaginal contractions and possibly a "squirt" in the female.

An explosion inside your body.

The best possible feeling … ever.

OOOOh yes! Yes! AHHH! Baby yes Baby yes yes! OOOooooh ooooh ooooh OOOH! Harder baby! Yes! Yes! YES! YES!!! Yes! YES! YES! Oh yeah! Your make me so fuckin' horny! Yes!

Take your pick. One or more of the preceding is the correct definition of "orgasm."

Direct G-spot stimulation produces waves of G-gasms. There are plenty of "doctors" that will swear there is no such thing as a "vaginal orgasm." These same experts will tell you that the only way to achieve female orgasm is by direct stimulation of the clitoris. Recent discoveries about the size of the clitoris - it extends inside the body - would seem to support my theory about G-gasms. The nerves of the clitoris pass through the G-spot and connect to the spinal cord for transmission to the brain cells. As the G-spot is stimulated, it grows in size. Somewhat like a beneath the surface penis. How awesome is that?

According to Elisabeth A. Lloyd, a professor at Indiana University, author of "The Case of the Female Orgasm: Bias in the Science of Evolution," published by Harvard University Press, there is a large percentage of women that never reach orgasm during intercourse. Lloyd goes on to say that there are women who **never** reach orgasm. Period.

Well, no shit. Unless you have a curved dick, it is almost impossible to stimulate the G-spot effectively during intercourse. A penis is not designed to stimulate the G-spot. Rather the function of the penis is to deliver sperm as close to the cervix as possible. Forget the missionary position, you will never hit the G-spot successfully – try doggy-style – you'll find the angle is better.

You are about to learn how to "wake up" the G-spot and make it explode. The method for G-spot stimulation you are about to learn will produce G-gasm after G-gasm. Again, a G-gasm is an orgasm achieved through direct stimulation of the G-spot not from the stimulation of the clitoris that is on the outside of the vagina.

What and where is the G-spot?

Back in 1950 there was a doctor Ernest Gräfenberg, M.D., who wrote the now famous article "The Role of Urethra in Female Orgasm." The article gets a little technical, but here are some excerpts of the important points that are relevant to G-gasms.

> "A rather high percentage of women do not reach the climax in sexual intercourse. The frigidity figures of different authors vary from 10-80 per cent and come closer to the statistics of older sexologists. Adler (Berlin) concluded that 80 per cent of women did not reach the sexual climax. Moosean guessed that 50 per cent suffered from frigidity, while Kinsey found it to be 75 per cent. Hardenberg's figures have a very wide range from 10 to 75 per cent."
>
> "An erotic zone always could be demonstrated on the anterior wall of the vagina along the course of the urethra."
>
> "Analogous to the male urethra, the female urethra also seems to be surrounded by erectile tissues like the corpora cavernosa. In the course of sexual stimulation, the female urethra begins to enlarge and can be felt easily. It swells out greatly at the end of orgasm. The most stimulating part is located at the posterior urethra, where it arises from the neck of the bladder."

"If there is the opportunity to observe the orgasm of such women, one can see that large quantities of a clear transparent fluid are expelled not from the vulva, but out of the urethra in gushes. At first I thought that the bladder sphincter had become defective by the intensity of the orgasm. Involuntary expulsion of urine is reported in sex literature. In the cases observed by us, the fluid was examined and it had no urinary character. I am inclined to believe that "urine" reported to be expelled during female orgasm is not urine, but only secretions of the intraurethral glands correlated with the erotogenic zone along the urethra in the anterior vaginal wall. Moreover the profuse secretions coming out with the orgasm have no lubricating significance, otherwise they would be produced at the beginning of intercourse and not at the peak of orgasm."

"The erotogenic zone on the anterior wall of the vagina can be understood only from a comparison with the phylogenetic ancestry. In the most commonly adopted position, where "the lady does lay on her back," the penis does not reach the urethral part of the vaginal wall, unless the angle of the erected male organ is very steep or if the anterior vagina is directed towards the penis as by putting the legs of the female over the shoulders of her partner."

"The anterior wall of the vagina along the urethra is the seat of a distinct erotogenic zone."

Dr G was one smart dude. I like my analogy better of a beneath the surface penis. The clit is the only visible part of a women's underground penis with the rest of it being beneath the skin.

Thirty years later, Dr. Grafenberg's work was resurrected, the now famous spot he talked about in his article was christened the Grafenberg spot or G-spot for short.

The G-spot is located about 2-3 inches inside the vagina on the outside or anterior wall. That is it – no mystery, no nothing – that is the G-spot. It is not like the lost city of Atlantis or some beautiful, secret area run by the CIA. You can imagine your partner's G-spot as almost opposite her clitoris but below the surface on the inside anterior wall of her vagina. When you have felt your way around in the vagina, you'll get to know the G-spot, as "bump" surrounded by the smooth fleshy anterior wall. The "bump" will feel ribbed, almost like the roof of your mouth. Memorize the first sentence of this paragraph.

When you have some time, perform an Internet search for the keyword – G-spot – look through the search results. You find articles from respected professors, so called authority magazines and publications about *"The G-spot supposedly is a small, highly sensitive area on the anterior (front) wall of the vaginal."* Or you find questions from some poor guy asking about female ejaculation ...is it real? Is it dreaming? It's sad when some of these doctors are still standing around scratching their ass and wondering where the hell they went and hid that damn G-thang.

Can you imagine, a bunch of supposedly educated gorilla doctors sitting at a bar discussing the existence, or non-existence of the G-spot? All they have to do is find a willing partner, arouse her, stick a finger in her pussy – and there it is – about two to three inches in, on the anterior wall. Hmmm ….

Ladies, you should not feel too bad if your man is a tad dumb when it comes to your bodies. Number one, there are no universal "owner's" manuals taped to anyone's ass and #2 it seems that some of the best sex researchers in the world wouldn't know your clit from your ass if it weren't for your titties being where they are!

Occasionally I get e-mails from couples that are not able to find the G-spot. The first piece of advice I give, is for the lady to get sufficiently aroused before her partner goes poking around looking for the G-spot. Whatever gets her going - watch a steamy x-rated movie, read a sexy story, talk dirty to her, tie her up, etc. Once her love juices are flowing – then it's show time.

An un-stimulated G-spot is only about the size of a pea and feels kind of like a dry roasted peanut shell. As the G-spot gets aroused and stimulated it swells to the size of a small walnut, giving you the clue that you not only found the spot but that it likes you! When the spot has swelled, the woman is in the big O zone and with more play; you will make her body sing.

In technical terms, the G-spot is a bundle of

nerve clusters that trigger natural painkillers within a woman's body. These painkillers are the same endorphins that release during childbirth. The nerve endings are concentrated beneath the surface of the skin in a protective bundle, which allows for sensitivity and ability to handle fondling.

Ladies, I recommend you experiment and explore your body. Learn where your hot spots are before you let your lover explore. This way you can advise him (or her) where those spots are and what to do with them. Not finding the spot and not knowing what to do with it can lead to frustration and disappointment.

To find the G-spot, place one or two fingers inside your vagina while you are squatting. Put your finger in a fishing-hook position and rub. Some women find it useful to press against the lower abdomen in order to ensure better contact to the G-spot. When the G-spot is swollen, your outside hand can feel it pressed against your inside fingers.

You will be able to stimulate your G-spot yourself; the problem with stimulating solo is that you run out of steam. You will be able to make yourself G-gasm several times, but eventually you will become a puddle, out of breath and exhausted. With a FB, you do not have to worry. Your FB can keep going long after you are unable to continue from complete fatigue.

Men, first as stressed earlier, get her sexually aroused. Don't ever stint on foreplay. Yeah, I know that you want to jump right in and get your fingers wet. Take your time; get her going first.

To locate the G-spot, face your FB while she is lying on her back and insert your index or long middle finger into her vagina. Then crook it upward toward yourself in a "come here" motion, sliding your fingertip along the top of the vagina until you find an area that is rougher than the rest of the vaginal wall. Make sure you have your fingernails clipped short before you do this - sharp fingernails will definitely spoil the moment. This rough or slightly ridged area is the G-spot, and touching it the first time, will often cause a woman to react with surprise and pleasure.

Second Base – The G-gasm Method

OK, does everybody know where the G-spot is?

One more time – everybody together: The G-spot is located about two to three inches inside the vagina on the outside or anterior wall.

Thank you! Very good, - let's ride!

Now that we know where it is – it is time to have some fun. I have had great success with this Method; the most important thing you can remember is that every woman is different. No woman has the same attitude towards this type of play. Take it easy – relax, have fun and make it fun for your partner. Communication is key; encourage her to talk.

Surprisingly, many sex manuals do not teach or even talk about direct G-spot stimulation and G-spot orgasms. Everyone has heard about and knows about the G-spot; yet many researchers and so called experts, still refer to it as the "elusive" or "mythical" G-spot. Trust me, the G-spot is where I told you it is. Guys, I know that some of you will want to guard this Method as a secret, so that you get all the chicks, but please;

help spread the word. There are plenty of women out there that need satisfying. Soon, you will be able to satisfy any woman, any time and give her as many G-gasms she wants.

Despite both spots offering the ability to create mind blowing orgasms the G-Spot is very different from the clit. In the beginning, you might treat the two in a similar fashion with some soft touching and light rubbing. However, when you have stimulated the G-Spot enough to get it going, that is when the real fun begins. A good guideline to remember will be to show the clit some mercy but to be merciless when it comes to the G-Spot! Within reason, most women will appreciate a harsher approach to the G-Spot.

Back To Gloria ...

You remember Gloria – she was my little FB tied face down on my bed with her pussy dribbling wet.

Gloria's ass was still wiggling up in the air. I reached between her legs and stroked her sweet pussy a few moments. Her pussy was dripping with excitement and her whole body was trembling. I then stuck my thumb into her hot little hole. With my thumb, I reached around until I found what felt like a soggy walnut.

"That's it – that's the G-spot," I thought to myself.

I started to rub it back and forth with my thumb. Gloria was going insane. Her ass kept twisting and squirming back towards my hand.

Gloria let out a gasp and moaned, "Oh my God ... that is unbelievable. A little to the right ... ohhhh yeah. That's the spot."

She was gyrating and moving like her pussy was on fire. I kept at it, back and forth with my thumb, then in a circular motion, then back and forth again. Gloria was going crazy; She was also going to explode soon. Her pussy muscles were clenching and pushing back against my thumb – she was losing it.

She was starting to cum, and was enjoying herself totally. She was encouraging me, as I moved my thumb with even more drive. I really got into it. Her legs clamped tightly around my hand and she lifted her ass off the bed as she gave a loud, drawn out, moan. She was totally out of control, and in the throes of a G-gasm – a huge one – and she wanted my thumb to press harder against her sweet spot. I kept my attention on the little walnut, careful to keep up the stimulation so I could prolong her peak as long as possible. She could take no more, she started to cum hard, pushing back up against my hand. Her G-gasm was as intense as it was long.

"OhhGawdyesSSSSSS...YESSSSS...," Gloria moaned.

"That was unbelievable," mumbled Gloria.

I gave Gloria a minute of two to catch her breath – then again started to rub her G-spot with my thumb. We continued on that way for about an hour. At one point, Gloria turned her head to look at me; she had this look of excitement, panic, shock, fear, thrill and exhilaration, almost as if she did not know what was going on. Gloria had about 10 mind blowing G-gasm's. She was a puddle, physically and mentally.

"Holy fuck … what the fuck? How did you do that?" Gloria asked, totally dazed.

I untied her; she got up to go to the bathroom and her knees buckled. She was shot – more than a puddle – she was a lake.

After a short nap, she asked, "What did you use on me?"

Sex is like a poker game; you need a good hand to win.

Gloria thought that I was using some kind of a battery-powered toy. She did not realize that my thumb did all the action. I kind of leaned back and made it appear that I did that to all my woman. In reality, that was the first time I had implemented the G-gasm Method that I had formulated from all the research I had done on the G-spot.

We spent the next few sex sessions perfecting her G-gasm experience. We wanted to see how many G-gasms she could stand without needing to stop and got to around 50-something in a five-hour sexual marathon. Since that time, I have seen some naturally multi-orgasmic women handle as many as 100 G-gasms quite well. It all depends on the woman. The farther along we went the more comfortable and knowledgeable about the process Gloria became.

From that moment on, I knew what I needed to know to have a full sexual experience. I have never been with a woman that did not find enjoyment, intense enjoyment at that, from an orgasm like this. Some have been able to sustain more G-gasms than others have, but all of them have had a wonderful and enjoyable time.

"Why don't all guys know how to do what you just did," Gloria asked.

"Well, guys don't get a manual on how to please women at birth, ya know?" I said defensively.

"You ought to write that manual," she said.

I am going to teach you how to please a woman. You will make her cum like never before. Kissing is nice, sucking their breasts is nice, nibbling on their clit is nice but you are going to learn how to give a woman G-gasm after G-gasm.

My partner(s) have blown their minds to a level that they never believed possible. The intensity, number and duration of both arousal and orgasms have increased exponentially compared to traditional and so-called "tantric" techniques.

While I have had great success with the Method, the most important thing you can remember is that every woman is different. If you move into dating and sexual types of relationships assuming that all women are the same, you are going to be mistaken. No woman has the same attitude and anatomy. While their anatomy may indeed be similar, they are not all the same, not by a long shot, and good communication is the cornerstone of great sex.

Later on, we will discuss variations of the basic G-gasm Method. Some of these variations will work better for you than others and will bring different results with various women. Some women will not have any huge orgasms but they may enjoy the intimacy and still receive enormous pleasure. Again, it just depends on the woman. Either way, plan to spend the first evening exploring her body.

Prepare your hands for this erotic experience. Scrub your hands well. Long manicured fingernails may look good, but not for what you are about to do. Keep the nails short and filed smooth. Before you begin the activities, to help prevent rough, dry hands in any weather, be sure to routinely massage your favorite hand cream thoroughly into your hands. The massaging action stimulates blood circulation throughout the hands and promotes the absorption of conditioners into your skin. Apply your cream often, especially after washing your hands or after submerging them in water. FBs will really appreciate your prep work.

There are only two actual "rules" for the G-gasm Method.

Rule number one is to have the lady use the bathroom before you begin. Stimulation to the G-spot will give her the sensation that she needs to urinate. However, if she knows she just did, it is less likely to bother her. The urination sensation does not last for a long time, though you don't want to end up having a stream of her urine land on you. You water sports guys might not mind this, it would be a deal breaker for most!

Set the mood. Some candles and sexy music really set the tone. Barry White has some music to G-gasm by. Barry White's impossibly deep and sexy voice, one of the most recognizable in music and his satiny love songs will bring any woman to her knees. Although after a while, her screaming with joy will drown out any music.

Rule number two is probably more important than rule number one is. Start with foreplay – kissing, touching, a back rub – whatever the two of you are in the mood for. Do everything you normally would do to turn her on, do not go directly to the G-gasm Method. This is essential; you must get her going first. This is especially important the first few times you attempt G-gasms. Lots of oral, dip your cock in her for a bit, try different positions, more oral and fingers and only then when she is about to burst, try the G-gasm Method. She should be fully stimulated and the whole vagina area engorged with her at the point of begging for more.

Some guys like to give their ladies an oral clitoral orgasm first, I recommend that you bring her close to orgasm, but don't let her cum. Use your talents and toys to bring her to the edge of orgasm over and over again. Many women are the one-orgasm types; their bodies are trained and are satisfied after one orgasm. Skip the clitoral orgasm; make her desperate for release. If she is moaning, dripping wet, and almost incoherent she wants to cum so much, now is the time to go G-spot thwacking full-time.

Have her lay on her stomach with her rear up in the air and her face leaning against some pillows. Make sure to have her legs at a comfortable width apart. Put a couple of pillows under her hips to get her tush up in the air. Position yourself at her side or between her legs.

Insert your thumb, thumbprint side down, in her pussy. Press the thumb downwards so that you are pressing towards the pillows under her hips. You will find the G-Spot right about where your thumbprint is. I know it sounds simple, because it is! There really is nothing to finding the G-spot. Keep in mind everybody's body is different. If she looks, or says she is uncomfortable, back off for a while, go back to doing "comfortable" things. You can always try again later or the next session. The first time is the hardest – after that, it is easy to find and play with the G-spot – insert thumb, press down (this is with the lady on her stomach, butt up).

Feel around for a smallish, rough bump that is bigger than a pea. The size will depend on the woman and the amount of foreplay. As she becomes more and more excited and the G-spot is stimulated, it will grow in size to about the size of a walnut. The G-spot is going to feel rougher than the smooth texture of the inner vagina walls.

Now that you found the spot, start rubbing. Start to rub in a back and forth or side to side motion. At this point, the key thing to remember is not to rub it too hard. You will be able to feel the spot thicken and grow against your thumb. Once this happens you will be able to increase your movement and get rougher with it. Rub it, as if you are trying to get a stain off your jeans.

Any guy that treats the clit rough will usually get a kick in the balls. After a clit stimulated orgasm, be it manually or with the tongue, even look at her clit and a woman will push you away. The G-spot is different. Once triggered and excited, do not treat it as a clit. In the excited state, the G-spot likes abuse – treat it rough. Beat an engorged, fully eager penis with a hammer and a man would say, " Wow – that feels great." The G-spot is similar. Be gentle with the clit – be rough with the G-spot.

As the G-Spot continues to swell, she will get the feeling that she has to urinate. However, that was the reason for having her take a pee before hand. I always ignore the request. The feeling will go away in a little while.

When the G-Spot gets excited and swells, it puts pressure on the bladder giving the woman a sensation of needing to tinkle. This feeling only lasts for about 30 seconds, and then subsides. Many newbie women become uncomfortable at this point; I assure you the feeling will change to a highly sexual pleasurable feeling.

While many women don't have to be asked to talk, and are more than willing to tell you how to rub their G-spot, I have been with just as many who need that little extra push to talk. To find out if you are in the right spot, just ask. You may find she wants you to move to the left or right. She might want you to be rougher and faster or slower and softer. Try rubbing side to side, up and down, "punch" it, rub round and round, tap the spot like a tiny drum, poke at it like you are trying to push it, jab at it like you are trying to pick it up with a fork, press on it with no movement, bring out the dentist's drill, vacuum cleaner, or chainsaw ... whatever it takes.

After a few minutes you should hear the mind-blowing madness which will be your woman having a G-gasm. The first time I watched this I could not believe my eyes. My life changed with one G-Gasm! She'll be bucking and pushing against your hand with all she has, moaning and screaming, she'll cum so hard she may squirt all over your hand.

To be able to give a lover that much pleasure is the best feeling ever. After the initial bombshell, your lover will be subjected to even greater pleasure as you continue the G-gasm Method. That's why I wrote this book, to teach others how to discover and explore the G-spot - a guide - to delve into the world of G-gasms.

Not everyone will have quick, fast and successful results – some couples will have staggering G-gasms within minutes – other couples try everything short of sacrificing a goat - we are not the same. The couples having trouble need to be persistent and they need to persevere and eventually, after many attempts, they will be like "WOW – WHAT THE FUCK – THAT WAS AMAZING." Once the first G-gasm is unleashed, all hell breaks loose. Whatever the immediate results are, remember that getting there is 90% of the fun.

A word of warning for the guys: Never try this

Method with your lady sitting on your face. If you do not drown from the pussy juice, you will certainly have a broken nose.

Meet Thelma

Her lips slid up and down my cock slowly. I sighed. She was good at this, but why wouldn't she be? She was an older waitress and I was a newbie bartender.

Thelma was about 45, she had established crow's feet around her eyes, a push-up bra, her brown thick hair a little bit stiff from the years of hair dye, but she was still hot. And boy could she suck a mean cock.

I had girlfriends who sucked my dick but not like this. Thelma would pause her sucking to lick my shaft then tease my swollen head with the tip of her pink tongue. She would wink at me when she saw my smile, and then tickle one of my balls with her middle finger as she pushed her mouth back and forth on my dick. Thelma was Talented with a capital T.

Thelma and I first met about twenty-five years ago, and I remember it like yesterday. I'm actually surprised that I remember it so clearly – after all this happened in the '80's – we did a lot of drugs back then.

I was working as a bartender in a place called "The Gold Rush." My boss hired me as a trainee bartender, working the day shift, and this was my first time on the night stint.

At first, Thelma did not really strike me as being hot as much as her personality was cool. We worked together all night, her ordering drinks for her customers and me preparing them and placing the cocktails on her tray. Whenever she approached the service bar area, she would say, "Ordering ... **cock**tails."

She would always emphasize "cock." As I would get her order ready, Thelma would wait patiently with a cute little smile on her face. She reminded me of my girlfriend's mother. She always said she had to hide her mom when I was around, which was true because her mom was hot. She was not safe.

We closed the bar around 2 AM that night – or I should say early that morning. I lived close by, so I asked Thelma if she wanted to stop over for a beer and unwind a little before she headed home.

"Sure, I'd love to stop over for a **cock**tail," she said as she gave me a coy little smile.

We got to my place, I cracked open a couple of beers, and we sat down on the couch. After a little shoptalk, Thelma leaned over to me and moaned that she was wet and that I needed to, "do things to her now."

"Whoa ... these older woman do not mess around," I quietly thought to myself.

I was not about to argue. I reached over and started to unzip the back of her dress. She batted my hands away, saying that she could do it faster. She only had her black work dress on, and that was easy for her to take off. Her black bra was next and there she was, standing in front of me with only her panties on. I was still struggling with the buttons on my shirt; I was too busy looking at her. Her panties, black lace, so skimpy that the "how to wash" label was the biggest part on them; they were last to go tumbling to the floor.

"Rip off your clothes!" She laughed.

As she waited for me to get undressed, she played with her brownish-pink nipples. She rolled them gently in her fingertips, giving them a squeeze now and then. She moved one of her hands down to her hot little pussy. Her cute little bush, was trimmed to what I call a "landing strip" – shaved along the bikini line and both sides, with a neat, trim line of hair down the middle. It was awesome.

Her index and middle fingers traced her pink lips. She pushed open her entrance and slid her two fingers inside her burning snatch. My dick was hard enough to go hunting. This chick had me so hot, I could go out find a moose, and beat the crap out of him with my cock. I pushed and pulled off my clothes, leaving just my socks on because I wanted to get in her pussy as fast as I could.

Thelma sat next to me. With her two fingers still in her pussy, with her other hand she reached for my cock. She gave my pole a few hard furious strokes, then grabbed the base of my shaft and squeezed.

My cock was throbbing; a little bit of white cream escaped. "Ohh!" Thelma moaned delightedly and leaned forward to lick off the cum – "I love that." Then she started to suck and suck and suck. Her lips slid up and down my cock unhurriedly. Slowly, she raised her head, pulling her mouth up the length of my dick; at the top, she sucked hard again, swirling her tongue on the underside. I sighed, what an unbelievable blowjob. She was an accomplished cocksucker, but of course why wouldn't she be? She was an older, experienced woman.

Thelma removed her fingers from her snatch so that I could get my fingers into her hot little hole. Thelma liked that. She looked up at me and leaned over to kiss me. I tried to move back from the impending slobbering cum drenched kiss – thinking that I will not enjoy it. Her lips locked onto mine.

"You're cock tastes so good. How do you like the taste of your love juice?" Thelma asked with a sheepish grin.

I threw my arms around her soft shoulders and pulled her towards me. We fell back with Thelma on top of me, our lips locked together. I put my hands on the cheeks of her firm, well-rounded ass and pulled her pussy to my face. She started to grind her hips as I let my tongue part her pussy lips, tasting her sweet juicy pussy.

"You know, it might not be such a bad idea if I try the G-gasm Method on her while she's on my face," I hungrily thought to myself.

Why did that thought cross my dirty little mind? Oh yeah ... I know why. I was thinking I am going to be super stud – I am going to hook Thelma on G-gasms. Hell no - everything started going south.

Funny thing was, while I was tongue fucking her and thinking about it, she begged me to stick a finger in her hole.

I did not hesitate; I was about to drive her crazy. With my tongue lashing away at her clit, I first stuck my index finger in her pussy, and then added my middle finger. It was the perfect position. All I had to do was the "come here" motion; there was the G-spot, the size of a small walnut, ready for rubbing.

I started Thelma with some light back and forth rubbing action, then switched to opposite strokes similar to walking on her G-spot. She loved it. The more I stroked, the more she started to move her hips. Thelma was humping my face hard, but I did not want to stop, knowing how much Thelma was enjoying herself. As I rubbed and licked her, I could taste the juices flowing out of her.

I started getting scared. She was rocking on my face, oblivious that I was down there. "Hey wait a second, look down, there's a face down here," I was thinking. Before long, she was thrashing and screaming in G-gasm delight. When she finished bangin' my face, she pulled me up, then began to lick my lips in frenzy and kissed me deeply. She broke off and exclaimed, "I love the way my pussy tastes on you."

When Thelma regained her senses, I pulled her

off me and said to her, "Ouch! Shit! I think you broke my fucking nose!"

I jumped up to go to the kitchen to grab another beer. As I stood up, blood gushed from my nose. Instead of a beer, I grabbed the roll of paper towels to clean myself up.

"I'm sorry, I'm sorry … so sorry … I could not control myself … sorry," Thelma cried.

"That's OK …"

Well sure enough, next day I went to the doctor and he had to reset my nose. I had to wear a splint for five days – that was attractive. How was I going to explain that to my girlfriend?

Lesson learned, never go Moose hunting with your dick, and never do the G-gasm Method while your FB is sitting on your face.

The Next Level

After the first G-gasm, you can trigger additional G-Gasms within seconds to a minute. After she cums the first time, start rubbing again, just as hard as before. The G-gasms will happen repeatedly. Of course, each woman has a different tolerance for this, so you will want to watch it carefully. Some women cannot take the rigorous abuse of her body so often. If she cannot stand many G-gasms, don't worry, because as sessions continue, the need and ability to achieve multiple G-gasms seems to progress. You will have her experiencing 10, 20 or more G-gasms per session in no time! Again, do not be gentle – unless of course she asks.

When you have her at that point – DO NOT STOP. The whole idea of using the Method is that you can keep going. Wait until you see her reaction when you make her G-gasm for the first time.

Now that she knows the feeling, it will be easier and easier to make her G-gasm repeatedly. The way to really blow her mind is make her G-gasm like that for 30 or 60 seconds straight, and then give her a rest to catch her breath and then start again ... and again ... and then some more.

It is like finding the key to the vault. Her body will know what it feels like from then on. Marathon sessions will be fun, but "quickies" in mall parking lots, or before the kids wake up for breakfast are a scream too. Once the vault has been opened, reaction time can be almost instantaneous if she is horny and you have 30 seconds to get your thumb in there and give her a good rub.

Guys, this is much better than just FUN. Most women do not have any idea that they are capable of such sexual energy and multiple orgasms. After five or six G-gasms, they start to look at you with amazement. Like, "How the hell are you doing that to me?" I do not give them any mercy. I torture them with G-gasm after G-gasm.

Female Ejaculation/Squirting.

This lady is a freak of nature – "thar she blows … " http://g-gasm.com/female-ejaculation.htm. In my experience, most women do **not** ejaculate. I emphasize that because many ladies fear they have failed, even though they just had 30 or more G-gasms, but didn't leave a bucket of cum on the bed sheets. There are women that do ejaculate and there are women that ejaculate sometimes.

Like mirages, rainbows, shooting stars and other nature masterpieces, female ejaculation has provided amazement and controversy. Many woman and researchers believe that because the fluids expelled during female ejaculation come from the urethra, that really the woman is experiencing loss of bladder control. In other words – she peed a little.

Men take ejaculation for granted. It is the "runny-prize" of sex – and the source of your future heritage. The only conceivable purpose of female ejaculation is for pleasure – very intense pleasure at that. The G-gasm Method can produce ejaculation when performed on a willing partner.

In some porno movies, there is a scene where the woman is shown ejaculating a clear or milky fluid. Is it real pussy cum? Is it trick editing? Is it pee? That is a lot of questions ... I think it is real.

I did a lot of research on female ejaculation, or squirting. I studied videos of women cumming, and I have read scientific articles. Hell, I am man enough to admit it - I even picked up a copy of Cosmopolitan Magazine a time or two just to try to figure out how to please a woman.

The tissue surrounding the female urethra fills with blood during sexual arousal, as the penis does in men. This results in the tissue becoming firm to the touch. Researchers believe that female cum is produced by the Skene's glands. Skene's glands are located in the urethra. These glands are similar in makeup to a man's prostate gland. Female cum is made of prostatic acid phosphatase, the same chemical secreted by the prostate gland and found in semen, minus the sperm of course. Do you remember my "underground penis" analogy? This indicates that a woman's ejaculation is similar in composition to semen.

Woman who experience G-gasms also enter the wonderful world of "squirting." Not all women, all the time experience ejaculation, some experience it sometimes, some women never squirt. Most females have the ability to ejaculate, but often do not and usually squirting is a taboo subject and not discussed openly. When was the last time you heard of anyone discuss "depositing **her** load" over a few beers?

In the past, medical doctors told ladies seeking advice about bodily fluids that they are incontinent, rather than told they are ejaculating. That led to shame and humiliation. What girl would want to be known as a bed wetter? Instead of enjoying the ejaculation sensation, many women believed they had "golden-showered" their partner. Many men thought they had been "golden throated" while giving oral to their lady friend. Many females will admit to having had an experience where they believed they had "leaked" during sex. The feeling of ejaculating is similar to peeing, a shower of warm wet liquid and a feeling of release.

Guys, be prepared for the flow of ejaculate. If

you are into "water sports," this is going to be a huge turn on for you. Do not react like "what the fuck is that – did you piss yourself???" because that will make it embarrassing for both of you. It is a normal body function. Make the lady feel comfortable, or she will dry up like a mud puddle and so will your sex life. You laugh, but I swear, if she thinks she peed herself during sex, she will lose her sexual high completely.

Ladies, you will be amazed at the amount of fluid your body can produce. Up to two cups of expelled ejaculate can slather your sheets during a love making session researchers say. The amount varies, as does the force of ejection. Sometimes, the guy's hand will get soaking wet, and other times her spunk will bathe the soles of your feet. How awesome is that?

This is a new slant on the question of "who sleeps on the wet spot?" We are not talking about a small amount like a few teaspoons that us guys eject; we are talking about a couple cups of milkshake. The fluid can appear like watered down milk or can be clear.

Guys, a Few Guidelines

Most women can ejaculate but many do not. In the same way that all women can orgasm even though some do not ever achieve climax, be it through bodily or psychological blockage, or in-experience. Playing with her G-spot for hours at a time does NOT necessarily mean she is going to ejaculate. That happens with some ladies some times. Don't get bummed if it doesn't happen – she is still having G-gasms and having a good time. She doesn't need to squirt. Again, some women will squirt a little; some will gush a lot; some will not spray at all; and some will shoot sometimes.

Back when you were a young teenager and started to spank your monkey, it didn't take you long to produce a load of jizz. The climax in woman is much more complex, but once they start they do not stop. Unlike men, there is more to follow. Give her a few minutes and she will be filling up like a Hummer's gas tank. Each subsequent G-gasm will deliver a different volume of liquid in all directions and velocities. This can range from a trickle of one ounce to an almost a chaotic cupful. Don't worry about the juices drying up, there is always plenty more.

As a rule, guys do not care who they cum with. For the ladies, it starts with the partners being compatible. Ladies that do ejaculate are conscious of "showering their lover." Men could care less, and prefer to "shower" in a flamboyant manner, i.e. facials, in her mouth, on her tits, you know, we like to make it dramatic – "WHOA BABY –check it out, that shot went five feet and landed on the alarm clock!"

Ejaculate fluid is different from the normal "pussy juice" or "love juices." Love juices are a natural lube for the vagina that appears with arousal. Squirting or female ejaculation comes from the urethra or pee hole.

Since female cum originates and emanates from the urethra, the fluid is mixed with a little pee. Men cannot pee and cum at the same time.

When a man is about to ejaculate, the opening to the bladder closes, making peeing impossible. A woman on the other hand, (so to speak) is able to ejaculate and pee at the same time. Frequently that feeling of peeing and oncoming orgasm are confused. That is why I stressed earlier that your FB should use the little ladies room, before you start your sexual activity. You do not want your lady to think about peeing – you want her thinking about G-gasms and ejaculations.

Kegel exercises are a good way to help control the peeing/ejaculating problem. Spend about a month training your muscles. This has the added benefit of greatly increasing the intensity of your orgasms, as the vaginal muscles become very strong with repeated Kegel exercises. These exercises strengthen a set of muscles known as the pubococcygeus or PC muscles. They are the muscles that both men and women use to stop the flow of urine. They are also the same muscles that contract and expand during orgasm.

Ladies, spend about 15 minutes a day for a month strengthening these muscles until they are so strong you can put your finger inside your pussy and grab it so tight you cannot physically remove it until you relax the muscles. You will have unbelievably strong orgasms.

Guys, you should also do Kegel exercises to develop extraordinary powers of sustained sexual activity and the power to withhold orgasm. Once you develop your PC muscles, as you approach orgasm you will be capable of literally "turning off the hose." Not that you always want to put off orgasm, but it's nice to know that you can. All you minutemen out there pay attention – DO YOUR KEGEL EXCERCISES!

A typical PC muscle workout: Start with tightening the muscles for 3 seconds, then relaxing. See how many times you can do this before they become tired. Next, start doing sets of five strong squeezes. Start with only a few sets, as with any exercise, you will work your way up to more sets. See Appendix A for more details on Kegels.

Once you work your way to three sets of 30 or more squeezes, your PC muscles are probably healthy enough for most purposes. The best part is that you can do these exercises anywhere. Do them while waiting in line at the grocery store; do them while at work, etc. Once you are skilled at Kegel exercises, you should be able to do them without anyone else knowing what you are doing.

Getting your lady friend to squirt for the very first time is like obtaining a PhD in sexology. The building of the ejaculation feels like the desire to pee. As soon as the urethra starts to tingle, second nature kicks in and she contracts her PC muscles to stop the flow of urine. She must oppose the contraction and try to squeeze out, as if trying to pee. This is not an easy concept, in that contraction of the PC muscles will actually stop the ejaculation from building. As squeezing the base of the cock and thinking momentarily of Mickey Mantle's batting average postpones cumming in men, "squeezing in" postpones female ejaculation. "Squeezing out" instead of "squeezing in" is a major barrier for many ladies trying to ejaculate. Practice will overcome the barrier.

OK guys, you have been warned, don't forget to use the biggest towels you can find; you don't want your mattress to start smelling weird after a while.

Working the G-gasm Method

♥ Peeing - the subject of most emails. Make sure she goes for a good pee before you start your activities, so she knows her bladder is empty. She will get that "I have to pee" feeling as the G-spot swells with excitement. That "I have to pee" sensation precedes huge multiple G-gasms and puddles of cum. Help her relax and accept the new sensations, mix it up with a little oral, while you are "training" the G-spot. Often the first G-gasm will happen when she least expects it. After that, it is easy to "rinse and repeat."

♥ After the first G-gasm, give her a short 10 – 30 second break, this gives her time to catch her breath but not long enough for her to come down from her high. Then proceed with more rubbing – the same way you did for the first O. Keep doing what you were doing – don't piss her off – she'll poke a hot stick in your eye when you are sleeping. If she is seriously overwhelmed and does not want anymore, this gives her the time to let you know.

♥ You are in control of her orgasms; you can allow them to come full on, or hold them back. Once you make her cum once or twice, you can continue this cycle until she begs you to stop, or until she goes into an orgasmic coma of sorts.

♥ If the woman you are with has an active job, you might want to save this activity for special events and weekends. I can guarantee that she will be sore and have a somewhat hard time walking when the next day rolls around.

♥ If there is not an immediate response from the lady, take it slowly; work her with foreplay so that she is as horny as you can make her. Work her orally and maybe even with little intercourse, and then try the Method again. If she doesn't respond, go back to something else; get her near orgasm, then return to the G-gasm Method. You are in no rush – have fun.

♥ When rubbing, vary the pressure. Of course don't hurt your FB, but it takes a firm hand and fingers, and a surprising amount of pressure to produce a G-gasm.

♥ This will become addictive to her. It will make your woman feel fulfilled and confident.

♥ Many women have expressed to me that a G-gasm is a mind-blowing experience. Their entire body receives a sense of relief. If a woman has never experienced this, you may want to give her more than a minute between each G-Gasm. Wait until she seems to have caught her breath. Once she can breathe normally again, it is time for round two, three, four, or ten.

♥ Do not worry about the size of your fingers because like the size of your penis it is going to have little to do with the amount of pleasure she ends up receiving. Length has nothing to do with this. Instead, you will be concentrating on the amount of pressure you are using and not how much you are shoving inside her.

♥ Experiment with just slightly different positions of your finger(s). The G-spot is easy to miss, and if you are off just a bit the rubbing will still feel good for the lady, but won't produce G-gasms.

♥ Try edging, to increase the intensity just a little bit more; learn the flow of her G-gasms and stop before she has one. Start rubbing her and get her close to G-gasm, then stop. Give her a minute for a breather and then go back to rubbing. Leave your fingers/thumb inside her but do not move them. When you finally rub her off, she will be bucking her hips and grinding back on you like a stripper whore!

♥ If you have never experienced female ejaculation, it may appear that she is squirting something. Don't worry! It is not pee or anything. It is a good thing, especially for the woman! Some women become embarrassed after ejaculating the first time – they think they peed in bed – but it is not pee. With G-gasms, some ladies will ejaculate – go with the flow, so to speak. Bring a towel ... or a bucket. Guys remember, keep rubbing past the "I got to pee" feeling, she is ready to G-gasm!

We'll talk more about gushing later.

♥ Ladies, I know that you are going to try to do this Method on yourself. Many women have a hard time being able to create the proper level of necessary pressure to bring on the type of orgasms they could with someone else doing the rubbing. In order for you to hit your own G-Spot, you would need to slide your fingers inside yourself, and push them upwards and out; an awkward angle – maybe you could do it while squatting. There are some good toys on the market. Do a web search for G-spot vibrators at: http://tonightsthenight.net

♥ Water based lubes sometimes help. http://tonightsthenight.net

♥ Once the lady has achieved a few G-gasm sessions, her body seems to know what to expect and not all the foreplay has to happen to trigger a series of G-gasms. You can warm her up a little, insert thumb/finger rub and give her three or 4 massive G-gasms. It is a great way for a little quickie before she heads off to work. She'll be smiling and glowing all day long.

♥ Most women are capable of G-gasms. Barring surgery and birth defects, all women have the correct "plumbing" in place to make G-gasms happen. This doesn't mean that the Method will work on all women 100% of the time. A combination of factors prevents G-gasms from happening. Fear, being the biggest culprit. Fear of "being dirty," fear of letting loose, fear of urinating and fear of losing control – these fears can be overcome. But birth defects, a cesarean section, hysterectomy or other surgeries may make it impossible to achieve G-gasms.

♥ Sex is not about the destination but rather the journey. If she's enjoying it, keep it up. With time, you will make progress. I receive countless emails from couples saying, "doesn't work …," "we can't …," "it seems that …," or "didn't work." Later, all of a sudden I receive, "WOW … unbelievable." Don't get frustrated and give up … keep at it, you will not be disappointed.

♥ Ladies, spread the word on the G-gasm Method. Think about it, what would happen if you, who experienced the ecstasy of G-gasms with a knowledgeable partner, had to move on to a new partner who lacked the necessary skills to help you achieve G-gasms? The same old, same old would not be good enough. You would have to teach him the skills; you would pass on the knowledge to your new lover. Some guys will take offense, but sex and what you prefer is part of everyday life that you share with your partner. Hell, you might even schedule some remedial classes if he was a slow learner.

Third Base – Variations of the G-gasm Method

"MMMM... YYYEEAAHHH," Gloria moaned out, showing clear pride in herself for becoming so aroused from my thumb in her hole. "Jeez, this is so nasty, and I love it! I feel like such a slut," I heard Gloria whisper.

"You say that like it's a BAD thing," I laughed.

There are many different ways to use this Method. Having her bottom in the air – although that is a good thing – is not the only way to achieve G-gasms! The only thing that is going to limit you with this Method is your imagination.

You are introducing your lover to a fresh new horizon – you need to talk to her, because some things are about to change – you need to know your partner's wants and needs. I have been with women that loved G-gasms but emotionally just could not handle them on a frequent basis.

Losing Control

Keep an eye on your lady, especially the first few times you try the G-gasm Method. If your lover is used to being in control, then the total loss of control that comes with G-gasms may make her uneasy. She will still be able to enjoy herself, but women do lose control during these sessions. Some women get scared – scared at the intensity, frequency and total loss of control of the orgasms. Many FB's will ask you to stop until they become comfortable with the Method.

This is where you have to decide whether it is time to hold her down and proceed or to go on to other activities. Often when she is at the "scared" point, her G-gasm is seconds away. If you can force a few more rubs, she will have no choice but to cum, and then you can repeat the process. Always be loving, understanding and supportive to your lady, but don't always let her call all the shots. Sometimes, even if you are usually a pussy-whipped boy toy, this is a great time to slap her ass, pull her hair, tell her she's a slut and a whore and tell her to shut the fuck up and that you are in charge now. Pull this off and she will know the meaning of respect.

Say Hello to Lisa

Lisa, a petite blond with a cute little body, and I were at a friend's party. At the time, we had only been going out for a very short time, and hadn't yet reached second base.

I invited Lisa down to the basement to get away from everyone. We both had a few beers, and were feeling good. "Have you ever had a G-gasm?" I asked Lisa.

"G-gasm?" she asked, waiting for my reaction.

"G-gasms," I repeated playing dumb. "You

know, a G-spot orgasm," I explained.

Lisa tried to keep a blank face, hoping that I would reveal more information. Lisa and I had been going out for about a month, and our relationship was starting to become serious.

"I have never had an orgasm without my vibrator glued up against my clit," Lisa confided.

I snuggled closer to her, nuzzling my lips to her face and mouth. I planted soft kisses under her chin and drew her eyes up to mine.

"What do you think?" I asked with a teasing voice that made her smile. "You want to try?"

Lisa pulled me closer to her, and drew her mouth close to mine. Her soft lips pressed hard against mine, and my tongue parted her lips as I explored her silky mouth.

Her nipples poked out from her t-shirt. I pinched them playfully, causing Lisa to let out a soft moan. I peeled away her shirt. Her bra concealed her beautiful breasts. Lisa reached back, undid the snap and let me get a glimpse of her milky white tits. Her bra straps slipped off her shoulders and the bra fell to the ground.

I plopped her down onto the floor and straddled her waist. My hands moved towards her to caress her cute little titties. Her nipples grew hard as I pinched them playfully. She reached under my shirt with both hands, and rubbed my smooth skin. She tickled me around my stomach, and started to fiddle with my belt to loosen my jeans.

I leaned down to kiss her, as she was bucking her hips upward to meet the growing bulge in my pants. She felt hot, excited, tingling.

My hands left her breasts and started making their way down to her waist. She moaned as I unbuttoned her jeans, and tugged at the zipper. I licked a trail down her chin and neck, touched her hard nipples with my hot tongue, and made my way down to her bikini line. She glided her pants down her legs and kicked them off onto the ground. Lisa's underwear followed next, her sweet pussy exposed to the cool room. She had goose bumps all over her body.

With my tongue, I made my way down to her pussy.

"Oh, god," she whimpered, pushing my head into her cunt, moaning as I licked her tight opening.

I reached around her and grabbed her round cheeks, squeezing them and pulling her sweet pussy towards my face. She wrapped both legs around my shoulders and thrust her hips towards me. With my tongue, I hungrily reached into her pussy as deep as I could. Executing the best cunnilingus skills I could muster she whispered, "You are so great ... You are the best ever, you know that?"

"Yes, baby," I answered. "Now she's ready for some G-gasm action," I thought to myself. I smiled, my eyes focused on her snatch, I reached up to stroke her tits and give he nipples a firm squeeze to really get her going.

Her pussy was so hot and wet. I slid my finger down her slit and back up again, Lisa let out a little whimper. I let my finger dive right in up to the knuckle. I rotated my finger around in a circle and then pulled it out, positioning myself where Lisa could see me, I slowly licked off my finger. I liked the way she tasted; I licked my finger clean. Then I let my finger dive and dip in and out repeatedly.

Finally, I reached in, found the G-spot and gave it the ol' "come here" motion. Lisa was ready; her G-spot was the size of a nice plump pea. Inside my mouth, Lisa's clit was growing crimson with excitement, and the sweet bump of her G-spot was plump and bloated on my fingertip as her love juices gathered.

With my finger, I rubbed her G-spot spot, trying out different degrees of pressure and adding some variety to my rubbing. Soon, Lisa would lose control and then the sweetness would overcome her... she wanted it, yearning for the huge release to finish her off. Finally, she exploded. Lisa lost control and came all over my hand. I gave her 30 seconds to regain her composure, and then started rubbing again.

Lisa looked up at me with this look of pure panic and excitement – she was losing control. I continued rubbing. I felt her fingernails start to dig into my arms as she pushed her hips towards my inserted hand. I knew it was just moments before she would G-gasm again. I rubbed faster and furiously. Her moaning and thrashing was getting increasingly louder which was a turn on for me. "I'm going to cum!" She yelled. She started shaking as she threw her head back and screamed. "OOOooooowww," she shuddered and whimpered.

I removed my finger from her hole and replaced it with my tongue. Lisa was flowing with love juices. I reached in her pussy as far as I could. She was so sweet. I continued licking her until she started squirming again. I reinserted my finger and found her G-spot - swollen to the size of a quarter - perfect.

"No, no, no, not again," Lisa whimpered as she tried to wiggle away.

"Oh yeah, Baby ... one more time," I said as I started rubbing her G-spot with one hand, and placed my other hand over her stomach to prevent her from squirming away. I always try to make the lady submit just a little longer than she wants to.

Lisa started screaming and begging me to stop. She loved it and hated it at the same time. She loved it because it felt so good, but hated it because I was in total control. Unless you know there is real pain – give them one more when they tell you to stop.

You Are So Naughty

Add in a little BDSM activities during your G-Spot marathon – Olive's favorite. This will really heat things up. A few well-placed spankings with your hand or a paddle will do. In addition to this, tie her down and control how many G-gasms she has! What a nice little mixture – the kinkiness of a G-spot rubbing together with a little bit of submissiveness – awesome. Be careful, this might be too intense for some women.

"Don't you dare try and wriggle away from me – OK …WHACK … now you get another G-gasm!" I shouted, "You'll like it if I tell you to like it!"

Olive moaned softly. I did it again. Her pussy got wetter – my thumb was sliding like a well-oiled piston in her pussy. Olive craved some light spankings. She loved it, and wiggled her ass to encourage more. I spanked her even harder, watching her ass get redder and redder.

Up until a few months earlier, I had no idea about how hot spankings could really be. Olive changed all that. Olive was not her real name, to tell you the truth; I do not even remember her real name. I will never forget her though. She was a thin Mexican beauty with dark brown hair. Besides the hair on her head and her eyebrows, she did not have a strand of hair on her body – right down to her lovable little pussy. I think that is why I nicknamed her Olive. One day, Olive and I were in a bar having a drink and chatting.

"The other day I was at a spanking blog, as I read a few posts, my pussy got so fucking wet. Normally I would just masturbate, but something inside my head snapped. I thought to myself that it is time to stop reading and imagining, it was time to turn some of my fantasies into reality," Olive confided.

I was not very shocked that Olive was suggesting that I tie her up and spank her. I knew she was kinky and fucking horny as hell. Now, I'm a nice guy, I don't go around beating the crap out of people – unless of course they deserve it – so I told her I was a little afraid of hurting her.

Olive convinced me that this is something that she really wanted. We agreed to try it – total domination intrigues me. We finished our drinks, and headed for the local hardware store for some duct tape.

We got to my place. "How hard should I spank you?" I asked Olive.

"I don't really know. I have never done this. I guess hit me hard enough to really experience the sensation of my ass being on fire," Olive replied.

"How many spankings should I give you?" I asked. I had not thought about that.

"Let's see what happens. Keep going until either I can't handle any more or your hand gets tired," Olive replied.

"OK – cool. The "out word" is "uncle."

"What is an "out" word," Olive asked.

"A word you say, that immediately stops all activities. Just in case you are screaming "stop, stop," but really mean "more, more." When you say "uncle" that's it – no more," I explained.

Olive agreed that this sounded like a good plan. "Start light and work your way up," Olive advised.

No problem, I had some big plans for her. "Where and to what should I duct tape her," I thought to myself. My bed was just a mattress, no backboard, so that would not work. Looking around the den, I spotted the entertainment center. Perfect, I can run the tape around the legs and back to her wrists.

"Put your wrists together," I demanded. Olive complied, I wrapped the tape around her wrists and told her to get on her knees and lean forward onto her elbows. I stretched the tape around the entertainment center's leg, then back around her wrists a few times, then once again around the leg.

Olive was able to move her legs, but her hands and arms were completely restrained. Olive closed her eyes. I could tell she was very nervous, yet also very sexually aroused. I wanted to see if the pleasure and pain thing was for real. I rubbed her ass a few times until I could not take the anticipation anymore.

I lightly tapped her bare bottom. With each whack, my stroke grew stronger. Olive's body was starting to gyrate and rock back and forth. She was enjoying it … I was enjoying it.

"Wow this is incredible," I thought to myself. After a couple of hard strokes, I stuck my thumb in her pussy. She let out a groan. Her pussy was dripping wet. I could not believe it; besides spanking, I had not even touched her yet.

"Your clit is throbbing and that sweet little cunt is dripping wet, isn't it?" Olive nodded, her breathing ragged.

I started to rub her already engorged G-spot with one hand and continue to punish her with the other. Her pussy was flowing like a river.

Olive screamed in pain when I spanked her even harder. Finally, it was too much for her, and she yelled, "STOP!"

I knew this really meant, "GO!" So, I continued the rubbing and smacking. Olive was rocking back furiously – she was almost ready to explode. A few more slaps landed on her now red ass, she was trembling. She begged me to let her cum, "Rub harder, please, make me cum." She cried.

I whispered, "You ready to come baby?"

I let out a silent chuckle at my horny little FB. Olive let out a muffled scream of relief, warm watery liquid gurgled out from between her thighs. I leaned over and licked all the way up to her pussy, licking up all those sweet love juices.

I could not take it anymore. I unzipped my pants and let my now raging hard-on see the daylight. What a sight. I mounted Olive from behind and started pumping away.

I slowly pumped in and out, knowing how good this was feeling as my dick massaged her warm, slippery inner walls, especially the G-spot.

"Come on baby. Fuck me like you mean it."

It was not long before my thrusts grew harder and faster bringing Olive to yet another G-gasm. She wanted more. "Yeah baby. Fuck my little cunt. Shoot your cum inside me!"

"You like this baby girl." I moaned jamming my hard cock inside her.

"Yes. I like it! I like it! Keep fucking me – harder - harder! " She panted, rocking back and forth against me.

I teased her a little bit, slowing down, pulling out, then pushing in hard again. I gave her a few swift slaps on her ass making her fuck me deeper and harder.

"I'm gunna cum!" I screamed out.

"Yes. Shoot your hot load deep inside my pussy!"

Olive was ready to cum again. Her pussy was clenching down on my cock. She threw her head back, we both exploded together.

"You're beautiful when you cum baby." I whispered.

"Uncle," Olive said softly.

Edging

I discovered edging almost by accident. It was Spring break; all my usual FB's had plans. Olive went to Cancun, Gloria was at Daytona, Lisa was in New Orleans. I had always done Florida for spring break, which had become a little mundane. This year I wanted to do something else.

I received a call from a former girlfriend named Barbie. We had split up over a year ago. I had actually fallen in love with her at one time, but was over that now. Back in the day, we made some beautiful sex together.

Barbie called me at around eleven o'clock on a Friday night – she sounded trashed. We did phone sex. It was good for me. You can never tell for sure what was going on at the other end of the line, but she sounded like she was having fun. The next day she called me again and invited me to visit her in Los Angeles.

"Barbie, if I go with you, it's just as a friend," I teased her. "Last night was just jerking off. Don't have any false expectations. I am not sleeping with you."

"Yeah, yeah – I know ... last night was fun though, wasn't it? No blow jobs either. We are just friends - not fuck or suck buddies. No hooking up!" Barbie replied.

"Huh?" I questioned playing dumb. "What was that last thing you said?"

"Well sweetie, in a week you'll be skiing on the water instead of on snow wearing a parka."

"I'm not your Sweetie!"

"Yes, dear - just a figure of speech."

"Now, no hitting on me. Or getting me drunk and vulnerable," I shot back knowing full well that's what we were going to do. We were going to do sex, drugs and rock and roll – not necessarily in that order. "

"I'll see you Tuesday at the airport in LA."

I got to LA Tuesday night. Barbie picked me up at the airport, and after a quick tour of the city, we got to Barbie's house around midnight.

"How about a shower together?" Barbie asked.

"Uh . . . well . . . uh . . . yeah, love to," I replied, caught a little off guard. I didn't think she would be so abrupt and casual about it.

Barbie led me to the shower. I held on to her neck and looked at her in a new way, as we let the warm water gush down our exposed bodies. Soaping up a washcloth, gently she began to wash my body. She softly ran her soapy hands down my back. I pulled myself closer to her, feeling her hard, erect nipples pressed against my chest. I gave her a tender and sweet kiss. She moved one hand from my back down to my ass and the other hand to my nipples, and squeezed them firmly. Our kisses became more passionate as she began to massage my swollen cock. Her other hand pushed a soapy finger into my ass. I began to shake uncontrollably as she quickened the pace and wiggled her finger. I was not ready to cum yet.

Edging is the art of bringing yourself to the point of orgasm, but being able to hold yourself back. It takes some practice and you need strong PC muscles. As outlined in the "female ejaculation" section, Kegel exercises strengthen your PC muscles.

A typical regimen for a strong and healthy PC muscle; practice Kegels persistently – short sets in the beginning, then gradually, over months, increasing both the number of Kegels you do a day and the amount of time you are able to hold a series of very long Kegels.

When edging, build yourself up to the point of orgasm, then stop or switch to something less stimulating. Practice this while masturbating. The advantage of building up and stopping is that it pumps your entire system. When you finally do have an orgasm with this method, you will see what I mean. It is the most powerful thing you can do.

Most women usually take longer and need more stimulation than men. Bring your girl almost to orgasm 5-6 times, she will begin to shake and quiver, and will beg you to let her cum. When she finally does cum, she will cum like the dirty little slut that she is. Oh, and you too - you both turn into wild fucking animals.

"Let me get your back," I said. I turned her around, took some soap from one of the wall-mounted canisters and lathered up. I started rubbing her back. Barbie closed her eyes, tilted her head back and told me how good it felt.

I pulled her towards me, as I reached around and cupped her breasts. I worked my way down between her legs, then ran my hands back to her nice rounded white ass. Barbie kept her eyes shut, her arms up in the air, and moaned in a sensuous, relaxed tone.

"That feels so nice," Barbie said with my hands gliding over her slippery skin, glistening and wet. My erect penis slid up against her ass and settled between the cheeks – almost as if it was mean to be there.

Barbie turned sideways to rinse off the soap. My hands continued to stroke her, one on her shoulder and breast the other moving down over her stomach and hips, the feelings tantalizing yet gentle. I slipped my soapy hand into the crack of her ass and my other hand between her legs. I could feel her pussy juices starting to flow, making her hot and wanting for more. Her twat was steamy with excitement; Barbie spread her legs just a bit to give me better access.

I slipped a finger in her pussy with my thumb pressed against her clit - she shivered unexpectedly. She arched her back slightly to get a better position. Barbie encouraged me by stroking my throbbing cock vigorously.. "Mmmmm," she moaned to spur me on.

Standing at her side, my fingers had a perfect angle to reach her G-spot. Barbie's G-spot was the size of a dime - she was ready. In her love hole, I gently inserted a second finger. The fingers in her pussy plunged in and out setting a rhythm that had her hips moving, my thumb gently caressing her engorged clit.

My other hand was busy working the back door. I gently inserted the tip of my finger inside her ass. Barbie groaned as the finger invaded her other hole. She pushed back on it, wanting to feel her ass stretch around it.

"Oh fuck, so damn tight," Barbie moaned as her ass deliciously squeezed my finger.

I thrust my finger deeper into her tight little ass, and she shivered as a wave of bliss flooded her body. She bit her lip as I finger fucked her ass. I reached to find her G-spot with my other hand. I started to stroke the now swollen love spot. She cried out with my fingers rubbing back and forth over her G-spot, my thumb massaging her clit, and around the other side of her body, a finger working her ass.

I could hear the sloppy sound of my fingers in her wet pussy, it felt so good – so obscenely dirty.

"How do you like that - You hot cunt! You little slut! Is this good enough for you? You like these magic fingers in your tight little holes?" Barbie could not speak, it just felt so good, all the while her hips pumping and gyrating.

"That's my little whore! You are a slut, aren't you Barbie? You love it, don't you?" Barbie loved it when I talked dirty to her.

"Oh hell yes!" she spit the words out from

between her clenched teeth. "Yes I am a slut! I am a whore, I'm whatever the fuck you want! Oh my gosh … I am gonna …"

I stopped rubbing her G-spot as she approached climax. I pulled my fingers from her pussy and brought them to my face, sniffing her juices before tasting them. Barbie stuck out her tongue and licked one of my pussy juice covered fingers. She loved the taste, and I sure liked what I was seeing – that really turned me on.

"Oh Baby give me some more …," Barbie whispered.

I reached back down to her love hole, it was slippery with cunt-juice and she swayed slightly as I inserted my fingers gently. Barbie spread her thighs wider and thrust her hips towards my fingers. All that mattered were my fingers. I started rubbing her G-spot again.

My other hand still working her ass, this time I rubbed her soaked cunt a little rougher than before. A muffled moan burst from her when my finger stroked her aching love button. Spreading her legs, she moved in rhythm with me as I drew slow and sensuous circles around her flesh.

I bent and kissed her once, twice, three times before sliding my tongue between her soft lips. She groaned with delight as she licked and lapped at my juicy lips. She started pulling and squeezing her nipples with one hand, and still had a firm grip around my cock with the other.

Her G-spot, swelled to the size of a bottle cap

as I rubbed it furiously. I could feel her squeeze my finger with her pussy and ass, "Oh, fuck, baby that is so hot … Oh, shit that's it … I'm done, I'm gonna cum…"

Again, I pulled my fingers out of her pussy; I wanted to prolong the first G-gasm as long as possible. I love teasing and playing by bringing the lady right up to the edge of G-gasm, and then stop rubbing for a few moments. After a few times of having her on edge, I will let them have their first G-Gasm. After the first one, you can expect a flood. Prolonging the first G-gasm seems to make the following ones almost intolerably intense and recur quickly.

Barbie kept riding my finger in her ass. She rode slowly up and down, doing her best to stick her ass out so that I could get more of my finger in her.

"Oh, god, that's good…," Barbie let out, "More, keep doing it … yes, give it to me …"

"Yeah you dirty little bitch …You like it in the ass --- don't you! Give me that pussy of yours bitch I want to make you squeal some more!" I continued.

My fingers found her G-spot again and I started rubbing - I was ready to let her explode. Her pussy started to shake and convulse. Her breathing came in shallow pants, as she started moving in rhythm with my fingers. Waves of pleasure crashed through her body, each one stronger than the last. Her wet walls squeezed my finger as it moved within her. I quickened the pace of me finger fucking her ass with one hand and rubbing her swollen G-spot with the other. It was more than Barbie could take!

She exploded into the wildest craziest G-gasm I had ever witnessed! It seemed to last forever! This G-gasm lasted for what seemed like several minutes! My fingers did not stop moving until Barbie's cries faded and the jerky movements of her body stilled. Wrapping my arms around her, I pulled her close, holding her tight. Her body convulsed so intensely I couldn't help but ask her if she was all right!

When done, she whispered, "Ooooh my GOD ... that was unbelievable ..."

It felt great to be able to give Barbie that much pleasure in completely new way. It's mind boggling for the woman, when she doesn't even know she can cum that way. It is especially incredible, because you can make her cum repeatedly using your finger(s). If your FB/girlfriend/wife tells you that she is not multi-orgasmic – prove her wrong; show her she *is* multi-orgasmic. Her reaction will be awesome.

Barbie and I finished washing each other, dried off and headed for the bedroom for a truckload of G-gasms.

Home Run – The Best Part

The best part about this Method is that after the first G-gasm, the carry-over effect is real and may last for hours. Most women can achieve another G-gasm with only a few well-placed rubs. Wait 10 seconds to 30 seconds, rub a little more and it would all happen again ... and again ... and again. That is what makes this Method so awesome.

Most woman experience clitoral orgasms, either by direct manual stimulation or oral stimulation. A G-gasm is like an orgasm on the inside. Guys, once you awaken the G-spot with your finger(s), give her G-spot some cock action.

Guys, try this ...

After a few manual – meaning finger – G-gasms, position yourself between her knees, while she is on her back. Spread her knees apart and hold her still. Make sure she is wet, or lubed up, and insert the head of you cock in her pussy. Instead of thrusting like a Chippendale dancer, rock back and forth gently, aiming your cock to stroke the top of her pussy. An upward curve to your dick, so it rubs right up along the top, or front of the vagina, makes the sensation for her even better. You might want to push her knees up and back towards her to get a better angle.

After a few minutes of this, she will slip into another world – maybe another universe. After her first G-gasm, she might appear to go limp - just kept going of course! Within perhaps 30 seconds, she will go into some scene from Psycho; she will buck uncontrollably. Hold onto her legs, you don't want her getting away, because you want to do it again, and again ... and then once more.

You have to try this method! After you do this to a woman, your confidence level soars to a new high. Your lovemaking ability seems to get better and better. Using this Method, with practice, you will be able to give her G-gasms almost on command.

Penis size doesn't matter; remember the G-spot is only two or three inches inside the vagina. You can have a three-inch dick and still massage her G-spot.

Gals, once you discover the "feeling" that his thumb or fingers make, climb on and work out the right angle for his cock to hit that same spot. You can make yourself G-gasm every 10 or 20 strokes until you either pass out or melt.

Instead of selling this book, I should charge per G-gasm. There would have to be some kind of "try before you buy" system, you know, like with software.

After you awaken and warm up the G-spot, with a G-gasm or two, stimulate the G-spot via penetration. In other words, warm her up and fuck her.

Back to Barbie ...

Barbie and I stood next to the bed, quickly dropping our towels and becoming a heap of flesh, kissing and fondling each other passionately.

I bent one of her pillows in half and stuck it under my ass to lift my cheeks from the surface of the bed. What this does is it lifts your hips up and puts your cock at an angle to where the lady can hit her G-spot. In order for her to do this, she has to lean towards you and then go at it. This allows the penis to keep passing over the frontal wall of the vagina, where the G-spot is located.

Barbie got on top of me and positioned herself over my cock. She rocked her hot, wet pussy against my throbbing member. She closed her eyes as she lowered herself down on top of me. She braced her hands on my chest, and did sort of an "ocean wave" with her ass moving it in small circles. Soon after she started riding me, she let out a yelp as her pussy quivered around my dick.

I was hitting her G-spot, because every in-stroke caused another squeal of delight. She arched her back and screamed to the ceiling, "Your cock ... it's making me cum ... I'M CUMMING ... I'M CUMMING ..."

Barbie went on gushing for like 45 seconds. When she finished, I guided her off me and positioned her on all fours.

"I love to bang your pussy. I want to bang it. So hard that you scream out my name. Do you want this big cock in your wet juicy cunt? You like that?"

Besides your now magic fingers, G-spot stimulation works best in the doggy-style position. On a psychological level, I think doggie style makes a woman feel... dominated and overpowered...almost a bit slutty... if that makes any sense. It is a "guy" position, very dominating and animalistic, you know what I mean? Most girls love it when pumped from this angle, because unless you have a banana for a cock, it is the best way to hit the G-spot with your tool.

Ask your FB to prop some pillows under her hips, face down. Stand or kneel higher than her ass, and thrust downward and along the front wall of her pussy, if you have a very smooth cock you might want to wear a French tickler condom.

"I love it when your large balls hit me from behind," Barbie said, as she positioned herself on her knees and elbows arching her back to lift her ass high for me. I loved her ass, which she thought was excessively big, but she loved the fact that I enjoyed grinding against it. This put my cock in the perfect position to hit her G-spot.

My thick cock plunged in and out of her; her pussy stretched out and clenched my dick. She felt so sweet. From this angle, each time I pushed into her, my thick head rubbed against her G-spot. Barbie was completely under my control … and loving it. The thrusts became rapid, leaving Barbie little time to recover between them. With one extremely hard push, Barbie felt her entire body erupt in the most all consuming orgasm she had ever experienced in her life. There was not a cell in her body that didn't feel awesome. I owned every part of her at that moment.

G-gasms feel like ...

Gloria, Barbie, MarMar, Thelma, Lisa, Roche, Shuga, Kat, Olive, Blondie, and others that have experienced G-gasms, have described them as:

"It felt like I had not come in three years, and was finally letting the entire year's worth of tension flood out of me at once."

"I completely lost all control of my body."

"A huge gush flowed out of my pussy – like in a porno film."

"Heavenly ... went on and on and on ... one long, continuous full-body orgasm. <Big sigh> ... I miss it already."

"One G-gasm, then another, another ... one after the other. I was amazed. I actually got terrified because I was out of control. I mean ... these orgasms were so different and intense from anything I had ever experienced. It wasn't local – meaning just in the vagina area – the G-gasms washed over my whole body."

"I have no idea how many G-gasms I had. When the G-gasms are happening, I couldn't tell you my name – never mind trying to count.

Explosive, intense, very wet, throbbing, blurred thoughts, taut muscles, murmuring, shaking, white lightening, twitching for hours – those are some words to describe G-gasms."

"G-gasms are not ordinary orgasms – more like body orgasms that last, roll into one another and move me to another planet. Steady vigorous stimulation is the key and DON'T STOP (especially when I tell you to stop)!"

"I have never squirted like that before - wow wow wow.... very different kind of release."

"G-gasms are awesome ... I worship your thumbs ... I am addicted to G-gasms ... I better insure your thumbs."

"Still walking funny." <Olive said this ... she's a riot.>

Email ... We Get Email

I love e-mail. Please send me feedback on the contact form at: http://g-gasm.com/ I am constantly learning new tricks and am more than willing to help the couple that is having trouble achieving G-gasms.

The web site also has a discussion forum for anything G-gasm related. Please visit and post your questions and comments. Help spread the word. Millions of ladies need G-gasms. The G-gasms are coming ... the G-gasms are coming!

"Wow, this is better than fun!"

"I am a middle-aged man in a relationship with a woman around my age. We have been together for a few years. While she is willing and able to accommodate me sexually, she usually does not reach climax.

I felt like I tried everything to make her orgasm, then I read about the G-gasm Method. I approached her about it and let her read your book. She was skeptical, but said we should try it. I had never tried this before so I spent some time warming her up – first we showered together, then a massage, then kissing and nibbling. She started panting, moaning and writhing around, getting more and more excited at my touch, I did not stop. I slowly started caressing her pussy – eventually inserting two fingers and rubbing the G-spot.

When she said she had to urinate, she seemed uncomfortable and wanted to stop. However, I would not quit toying with the G-Spot. She almost forced me off her, but then the sensation kicked in! She not only had one G-gasm, she had four! The rate and the frequency of G-gasms increase with each love making session. The most she has ever had in one night has been 17, which is so incredible!

Every chance I get, I pass on the G-gasm Method. I only hope it helps people as much as it has helped us."

Matt S.

RE: "Wow, this is better than fun!"

Matt, that is awesome. I think that the sensation of having to pee is the number one reason some couples have trouble experiencing G-gasms. Once she gets past that hurdle – it's ecstasy! Good work BTW with the not quitting.

"Tried it ... loved it"

"I knew from the moment I found out about this Method that I wanted to try it. However, as a single woman I did not know when I would be able to try it out. I tried with my own fingers but the positioning made it hard to reach. I decided to buy a G-Spot vibrator and had excellent results with that, but obviously, that is only a close second to a warm, masculine body. There is a big difference between a man making love to you and a vibrator giving you G-gasms.

I am writing this today because I finally got a chance to experience it first hand (LOL). Wow! I never imagined anything so fulfilling! I was lucky enough to meet someone that actually knew this Method, and laughed when I told him that I wanted to try it. He tied me down so that I could not get away and he spent the entire evening exploring my body. I had 25 G-gasms from G-Spot manipulation alone! This is not including the other orgasms I had that night.

This is fabulous! I do not know how I used to live with only one orgasm!"

Cathy L.

RE: "Tried it ... loved it"

Cathy – It is tough for you gals to succeed with the Method with your own fingers. You can reach the G-spot OK, but most girls cannot stroke with enough pressure to G-gasm. To increase the pressure, with two fingers in your pussy place the palm of your other hand on your abdomen right above your pubic bone - just below your navel and squeeze down with your palm, while pressing up and out with your fingers.

Great selection of toys at: G-spot vibrators.

Glad to see you found a FB.

"Disappointed"

"I have only tried this once but I have to voice my disappointment. Although we followed the steps properly, the Method did not work. We tried it while I was lying on my stomach and then on my back. We even tried it on my side. My partner tried soft and hard rubbing and though it felt good for a brief amount of time, I never got past the urination feeling.

I have never had any nerve damage or anything so I am not sure why this problem is occurring. We do know that he hit the G-Spot- any advise."

Shawnee

RE: "Disappointed"

Man, do you give up easy! You tried it all of one time and you're done. You'll be sorry … No, seriously don't give up yet.

I am guessing it has to do with poor muscle control. Forget about the Method for a few weeks. Start doing some Kegel exercises to strengthen you PC muscles – we talked about that in the book – this will help you get past that "I have to pee and am not comfortable" hurdle.

What is your lovers email address – I want to send him a note to tell him to make you as HORNY AS FUCKING POSSIBLE before he goes poking around the G-spot. This is especially important the first few times you try the G-gasm Method.

"How long should I rub"

"Thank you for this great information. Last night, the ol' lady and I were experimenting with the G-gasm Method. She claims that she has a big butt, (I love it just the way it is) so is a bit uncomfortable laying face down, with her ass up in the air. She propped herself up on one knee – almost at a 45 degree angle from her hips to bed. She lifted her leg a bit, and I inserted my thumb from behind.

She was hot, and came within 30 seconds. I kept rubbing, and she kept moaning as if she was constantly cumming for about 5 minutes. Eventually she went limp – I actually had to check if she was still breathing.

My question is – when should I stop rubbing? Thanks."

Tom the limo driver

RE: "How long should I rub"

Hey Tom –

Glad to see you guys having fun. I like to keep the G-gasms going in a rolling pattern. Build her up to a G-gasm, stop rubbing for a few seconds to a minute, and then start rubbing again. This gives her a little break, but not enough of a breather to let her down from her sexual high.

If she is in shape physically, you can keep her cumming for hours or until you get a thumb cramp (which you will get until you build up your thumb muscles). Mix it up a little – give her one huge 5 minute G-gasm, then add some mini G-gasms followed by a mother lode G-gasm, followed by some edging (bringing her to the brink of a G-gasm, but then stop rubbing thereby putting off the G-gasm), followed by the mother of all G-gasms. The power is all yours Tom.

Vary it up, add some toys, add some spankings (if she's been a bad girl) – try it different times of day or night. Your lady will appreciate your dedication to **her** pleasure.

"Shocking!"

"First off, let me start by saying that I do not know how to thank you enough. This Method has changed my life. My sex life was good before, but this is just ridiculous. We use the Method regularly and in many different positions. After he warms me up with his magic fingers, I get off by him doing me doggy style. Fun! This Method has turned me into a nymphomaniac for sure LOL.

The sensations are incredibly hard to describe. The feelings stretch from my toes all the way to the top of my head. My body tingles and I explode in pleasure. Once the first G-gasm hits, I am lost in the sensations. I reach at least 20 G-gasms per night, but have had many more when we have longer love sessions. I have had a chance to use this with more than one sex partner and it works with all of them – I leave your book laying around the living room table. Only problem is that some men are harder to train than others :o).

Thank you for sharing such a wonderful Method with the world. Now that I have learned how to master it I seriously could not imagine living without this pleasure in my life!"

Gail K.

RE: "Shocking!"

You are most welcome! When can I come over for "training?"

"I'm Trying!"

"My wife found out about your Method from some friends and could not wait to try it. I had no problem because I love to give her pleasure but our results are not as successful as I could have hoped. There was literally no sensation for her when it came to this activity. I tried for some time, but no reaction from her. She didn't even get to the needing to pee feeling. I wanted to be able to wow her with this but unfortunately I think I am one of the small percentages of men that just do not know what they are doing."

RE: "I'm Trying!"

Keep at it, don't ever give up. Remember, that all women are different. Some take a little longer to wake up the G-spot – but once it is awake – WATCH OUT! Do not make this out to be some kind of an experiment – weave the Method into your other sexual activities. You are not baking a cake; do not tell her you are going to try "something new." Don't act like a gynecologist, act like a lover as you make love to her G-spot.

Take your time making love to her. What is her "hot spot?" Does she like oral stimulation? If so, get her to the brink of a clit orgasm a few times. Do not let her cum; just get her close to climax. Get her a hot as fucking possible without her going over the edge.

When you see she is really starting to boil over, get her comfortable and face down over some pillows. Kiss her back, nibble her ass – you know, all the stuff you normally do – you do normally do that ... right? Get her to relax and gently work your thumb into her now drenching wet pussy. Star rubbing slowly and softly, as she gets more excited, increase the pressure and speed of your rubbing. She has to get used to the new thing that your thumb is doing. It does feel weird for her the first time; get her to relax and build her up slowly.

Once she G-gasms the first time, get rougher with the G-spot to keep her cumming for a long time.

"WOW"

"This was amazing. I am multi-orgasmic as it is, and it really doesn't take much to bring me to an orgasmic state. When my husband brought this information to me, we were interested in trying this to see how it would work for us. Things did work well. In fact, I will admit I had 26 orgasms that night in a span of the two hours we were messing around.

I pass it on whenever I can. I know many of my female friends are impressed with the results.

If the women were multi-orgasmic they state that it feels great, but they are not quite as amazed as the women that were used to only one orgasm per evening."

RE: "WOW"

Being a man, I can't even fathom 26 orgasms per night. I think my dick would fall off.

Being naturally multi-orgasmic gives you a head start on the one O per night girls --- but they will catch up! Enjoy!

NOTE: Despite having made this book primarily for a male/female audience, I received this testimonial from a female that used the Method on her girlfriend.

"Two G-spots are more fun than one"

"My girlfriend bought your book. We both read it, I have to admit I was a bit skeptical, but we decided to try it. What happened next is something I will never forget. It took us a couple of times to perfect the Method but it works well on both of us. Not only does one of us benefit with this Method we both do! We managed to work out a situation where we can have G-gasms together using either our fingers on each other or using a double-ended dildo.

This was the best thing that has ever happened to us. What is even more amazing is that before this I swore the G-Spot did not even exist. Neither of us had the pleasure of experiencing anything like it. Thank you so much for sharing this excellent information."

Shawna and Robbee

RE: "Two G-spots are more fun than one"

Oh my gosh … is it getting hot in here? Can someone please open a window!

Can I come over and watch one day? I swear I won't touch either one of you, just put me in a corner where I can watch. Enjoy!

"Still Working at it"

"It has been fun and exciting for me. At times, frustrating but you know what they say … practice makes perfect. Since my wife has started reading your book, she has become much more open about her feelings, especially during our love making sessions.

Thank you for the advice, we have both learned a great deal about our bodies and ourselves. Trust is not an issue – we have been married over 20 years and we spend 90% of our free time together.

I think there are some ingrained inhibitions floating around. We are working on them but still it has been a very pleasurable journey for the both of us. We haven't gone to the bank with any G-gasms yet, but you have revitalized our marriage and made us feel like stupid teenagers again just discovering sex.

WTF – I thought I knew everything! You rock – thanks."

Joe Deli

RE: Still Working at it

Joe D – Often I think of my own upbringing. My parents would never dream of discussing sex or even male/female relationships. There is no wonder that people have inhibitions hovering around the cobwebs of the mind. Did you or the Mrs. have a religious upbringing? Think of all the nonsense they teach there. These thoughts go way back in your psyche and sometimes need professional help – I always use my local bartender – he makes me feel better about myself … at least for a little while.

Good luck you guys … let me know how you make out. At least I turned you into horny fucking teenagers again.

"Who knew?"

"I cannot thank you enough! I have never had a very fulfilling sex life but my husband is a miracle worker when it comes to perfecting this Method. He has always been very patient and he sprung this on me, so I was in complete shock with what happened. He asked me to trust him, but I was nervous when he began holding me down.

At first it might seemed a little intense – with the have to pee feeling, but I worked through it. The sensations are so worth it, I can't even begin to explain. The first G-gasm hit me like a ton of bricks. He let up for a few seconds then attacked my G- spot harder and faster; I came so fast and so powerfully that I think I literary arched into the air. It was beautiful - total mayhem. He played with different angles with his two fingers, rubbing in all sorts of motions, teasing me, working me into a G-gasm, then stopping and making me beg. My current record is set at 15! Thank you so much for sharing this wonderful knowledge with the world.

When someone peels me off the ceiling, I want to buy you dinner."

RE: "Who knew?"

Awesome ... let me know when you get up to 50 per night.

"Can't get enough"

"I have told everyone I know about this fabulous Method! I tried it out the day I found out about it and have used it regularly since then. You are simply fabulous for sharing this information because women all over the world are now able to experience what they should have been experiencing all along.

My wife has never been more satisfied. She walks around all day glowing because she is so happy and relaxed. We are able to do this in multiple positions and with different angles. Each one makes her scream in a different way! We have not had this much sex since we were teenagers! Again, thank you so much. This is just great!"

RE: "Can't get enough"

Ahhh ... to be 18 again. I don't know if my body could take it ... do I get a fresh liver to replace the one in the wagon? Enjoy!

"New Position"

"Last night, I was on my hands and knees, my husband behind me, he inserted one finger, then a second finger in my pussy. This really got the juices flowing, but then he put his thumb in my butt. He was opening and closing his fingers and thumb like a mouth. I was shaking ... the bed was soaked ... he said he could feel it running over the back of his hand."

Maggie K.

Re: "New Position"

That's the beauty of the Method – there is no right or wrong way to perform. Do and try anything that intensifies the feelings – the more things you add to the mix the better.

I've tried dildos, extra fingers, two thumbs, veggies, tongue, talking dirty, nipple clamps, paddles (.....that wonderful line between pleasure and pain), restraints, porn – you name it ... I'll try it at least twice to make sure it's right. Just when I think I've reached the limit – I find a new ingredient.

My favorite position is lady face down, butt up in the air, insert thumb, rub and wait for the pyrotechnics to start. The great thing about using the thumb is that it keeps you from targeting too deep in the pussy and you can get a good hard rub going.

Autogasms

Many women and men have written in to talk about something amazing called an autogasm. The autogasm is a new phenomenon that occurs when the body is in a blissful state from receiving so much pleasure. Mini G-gasms continue for hours after any sexual activity has ended. A woman that is able to have them will never forget them.

I have never been with a woman that has experienced autogasms, but from talking to couples that have had the pleasure, they are a series of mini G-gasms that recur as the lady is coming down from her sexual high. In all cases, the love making sessions were long and intense, lasting more than two hours with the lady experiencing 20 or more G-gasms in that period.

Again, not all couples encounter autogasms. Imagine your lady going to work after a 20 something G-gasm session.

"Roche, why are you walking so funny?" asked Mr. Klumpkin, her boss at work.

"Oh, I don't know ... hubby and I were ... oh my gosh ... what the fuuuu ... oh man ... no way ... this is not ... oh gooooowwddd ...."

"Roche, what's the matter? Can I get you some water?"

"Towel ... please ..."

Guys ... A Warning!

This is a very powerful Method. You are the giver of great pleasure. Your lover may not being able to think about anything else but being in your bed ... you could call it obsessed.

The most important thing you need to remember is that every woman's body is different. The standard Method will not work on all women, which is why I provide multiple options and variations. One variation may work, while others will not. However, if you are showing them the time and attention they need they will often have a great time regardless of whether it works fully or not. There is no such thing as 'bad sex.'

Don't take this knowledge too technically and never treat the event as a "sex workshop" about being able to make a woman have that many orgasms. All that does is make it harder on you and less enjoyable for her. This is all about pleasing her. OK, you know you will get yours later.

I received this e-mail from one of my readers Matt S.

"My girlfriend Linda and I love your book – I'm perfectly happy stimulating her to the point of G-Gasm after G-Gasm. Our sex life has never been better.

The other day, I went on our computer, there was an open window with Google search results – the phrase Linda was searching for – "how to please a man."

Thanks!

Matt S."

As a willing partner, you will get yours. Trust me, she will want to please you as much as you satisfied her. You are going to hear this:

"Cum in my mouth ... I want to taste your semen."

"Cum in my mouth, honey," she urged. "Shoot a big load down my throat, baby. I want to taste it! Tickle my tonsils with your love juices."

"Oh my ... I ... I ... ohhhh yeah ...ahh ... yeah ... ohh ..."

You are entering a completely new paradigm regarding sex – a new way of performing and pleasing your partner. More than likely, you will be introducing her to her G-spot. She may have read about it, heard about it or maybe even played with her G-spot; what you are going to introduce, she has never experienced sexually. It is a complete change in consciousness, a new approach to sex.

You will reach a higher level of connection with your lover when she trusts you enough to let go.

Barbie described it to me as, "What a woman feels with the Method is hard to explain with words, unless you have experienced it, there is no way you can understand. Once you get past, the urge to pee you have broken through the last obstruction and given yourself entirely to your partner, who now must have your total trust. This lack of trust is a reason that some women do not experience G-gasms the way they should."

Many-experienced woman find this Method scary or uncomfortable. They have been used to controlling the destiny of their orgasms, and now they cannot – you are in charge.

Definitely, take it slow with a sexually inexperienced lady. Could you imagine, a girl that has been playing around with masturbation and here you come along and blow her away with 20 or 30 dripping wet, massive G-gasms. Take it easy, take it slow, do the stuff you should be doing first like necking, heavy petting before you start with G-gasms.

Guys, what exactly does this mean? This means, that this Method is all about her. She has to trust you enough to hand over the controls to her body, because she will be helpless once the G-gasms start. She must let go completely. She will be screaming "OH MY GOSH" until her throat is sore and eyes rolling back in her head. There is nothing ladylike about it. The first time, she could actually get scared.

If she is used to gentle rubbing and stroking, she will find that the G-gasm Method is much more intense and physical than a clitoral orgasm.

Oral sex for a woman is usually the best. Now you have something better in your arsenal. You can literally keep her going for hours until she hyperventilates or passes out. She will be thrashing and screaming.

The best part is afterwards, she will be glowing like a hot light bulb in a cold hard steel pot. Her self confidence will be at an all time high. Many women need that "loving" thing at the end of a G-gasm session, so they don't feel like they're being used or abused. They need to re-establish intimate contact and connect with you, kind of like being welcomed back from a long trip. Many soft kisses, embracing, caressing, you know guys - mushy stuff - that girls crave. Describe to her how incredibly fucking sexy and turned on you were, by watching her cum like that. She will feel even better knowing that you had a good time too.

You on the other hand, will be strutting around the room like a well-oiled porn star. You will feel like you are ten feet tall because of what you can do to her. Any kind of sex related problems you thought you had are now gone. Small dick? No problem you have your thumb. Premature ejaculation? Not a problem anymore; she will be satisfied way before the time you have to stick your cock in her. Can't get it up? No worries – your fingers are always ready. You are a living legend. You are God at the singles bars.

You get a tremendous sense of satisfaction knowing you have given your woman THAT much pleasure. It is incredible! It also gives you a feeling of confidence whenever you look at a woman and knowing what you could do for her even without taking your pants off.

Guys, you will know why it truly is better to give than to receive. The look on her face is priceless. There is nothing more satisfying than hearing her scream with pleasure, teasing her, and knowing that she is getting off because of you. Use this outline of the G-gasm Method as a roadmap to pleasure, but sometimes the most enjoyable parts are the detours.

This is an incredible Method to master, something you and your lover have to work on, to make her a multi-orgasmic, quivering, sweaty, sticky, convulsing, twitching mess every time you make love. Completely awesome. Enjoy!

Appendix A – Exercise

Hand

Forget about penis enlargement and premature ejaculation – those problems are in the past now. Your only concern now is the condition of your hands. The last thing you want to do is to have an awesome G-gasm session going on and before she can scream UNCLE, your hand cramps up. That's not good. Let's say you only gave her about only ten G-gasms and she wants and needs 30 or more. If your hand craps out, she is going to be pissed.

First thing to remember is that most everyone has two hands and ten fingers. If your right thumb is getting tired, switch to your left hand, if your thumb is getting cramped flip her over and use your fingers.

I've found that the thumb can last longer than fingers doing the "come here" motion, the reason being that the thumb is in a direct line with the larger arm and shoulder muscles. With the "come here" motion, all the movement is with you hand muscles, using your thumb, you use your thumb muscle, arm muscles and shoulder muscles.

Squeezing a hard rubber ball is a good method of hand exercise. If you want to spend a few bucks, get some handgrips with added weights. Start with small sets of squeezing, and work your way up to 100 hundred or more.

PC Muscles – Kegels For Men

Guys, here's a simple set of exercises that can bring back a firm erection, create mind-blowing orgasms, and gives you a healthy prostate. Strong PC muscles give you the ability to stop the flow of ejaculate during orgasm, thereby delaying and prolonging your fun. When you finally do ejaculate, you might splatter the headboard behind you.

Kegel exercises, also called PC exercises strengthen the pubbocoxygennus muscle or PC muscles. The PC muscle surrounds your anus and prostate gland. The PC muscle is the muscle that pumps when you ejaculate. Strengthening - and learning to control - this muscles is essential.

To find your PC muscle, start to urinate then stop in midstream. The muscles that stop the flow of urine and pump when you ejaculate are the muscles to exercise. If you have trouble stopping the flow of urine, you probably also have weak orgasms.

Do not exercise them while urinating.

PC clamps: squeeze and release, over and over. Start with "sets" of twenty, and build up to sets of 100 or more. Do these every day for the rest of your life. This is a great exercise while you are driving or standing on line at the grocery store.

Long squeeze: Hold your PC muscle compressed tight for a count of twenty. Build up the strength to 30 or 50 count.

Slow squeeze: Tighten the PC muscle as slowly as you possibly can – repeat as often as you can.

You can do these exercises anywhere and at any time, there is absolutely no excuse to neglect your exercises. No one will know that you are squeezing, unless of course you keep smiling like a dumb ass while doing them, thinking about the next G-gasm session.

Ever see porn star Peter North in action – you have to see his <u>cumshots</u>. Rumor has it that he does his PC regimen daily. You should too.

PC Muscles – Kegels for Ladies

Kegel exercises were originally created to help women strengthen their PC muscles, to help stop urinary incontinence after childbirth, when the PC muscle has been stretched out. The Kegel exercise turns out, has sexual benefits also.

Ladies, There are three reasons you should do your Kegel exercises.

First, a strong PC muscle will help you overcome the "have to pee" feeling during the G-gasm Method.

Second, with the PC muscle is stretched out, less of the vagina and G-spot area is in direct contact with the penis and therefore receives less stimulation – less fun for you and the man.

Thirdly, a well-toned PC muscle will give you a powerful ejaculation. Keep the PC muscle exercised with Kegels – you will have greater blood flow to this area, and the greater ability to become aroused and feel sexual pleasure. Want proof – check out these <u>squirters.</u>

The great thing about doing Kegel exercises is that no one knows you are doing them. While you can do all sorts of variations, the basic Kegel exercises are:

Contract your PC muscles. Hold initially for a count of five; build up gradually to a count of twenty. Repeat ten times and practice daily. Like with all muscles you are better off building the PC muscle slowly and regularly.

You can also add quick Kegels, contracting and releasing the muscle for ten seconds. Relax for a few moments and then do it again. Try a "rolling" Kegel with your PC muscle, squeeze only at the entrance to your vagina initially, and then rolling the contraction up the length of your vagina and back down.

Spread the word – let the G-gasms roll!

Please visit us online at g-gasm.com

www.ingramcontent.com/pod-product-compliance
Ingram Content Group UK Ltd.
Pitfield, Milton Keynes, MK11 3LW, UK
UKHW041412180426
11947UKWH00007B/85